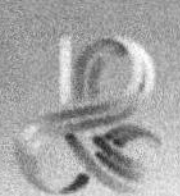

ILLUMINATE YOUR PATH
TO HEALTH AND FITNESS

BY RION DION

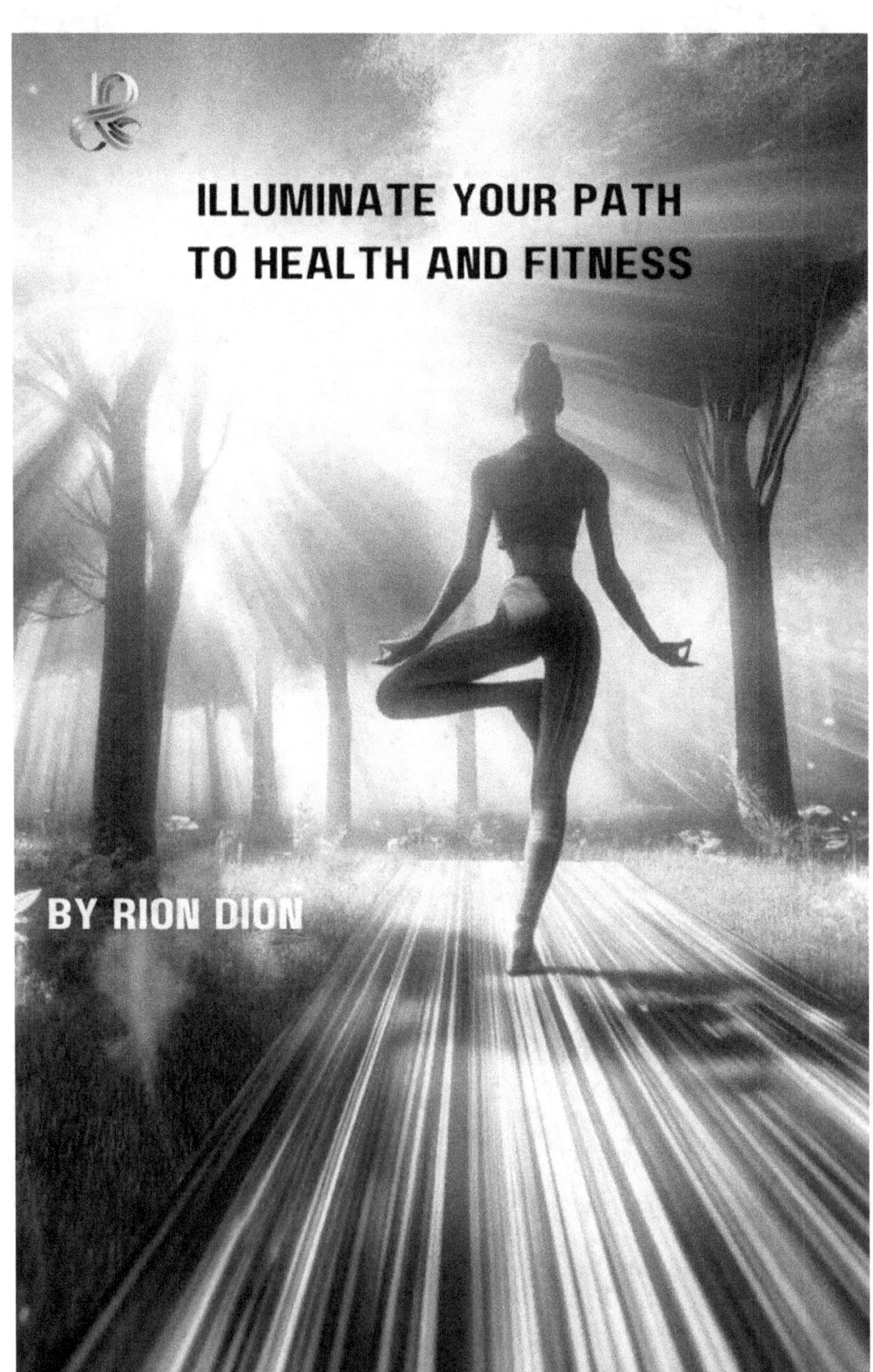

ILLUMINATE YOUR PATH
TO HEALTH AND FITNESS
BY RION DION

Table of Contents

Introduction

1.

Welcome to Lumeim: Introduction to the Brand and Book

2.

Philosophy of Lumeim: Ethos of Health, Fitness, and Sustainability Part I: Foundations of Fitness and Health

3. Getting Started with Fitness: Basics for Beginners to Advanced
4. Developing a Sustainable Fitness Routine: Building Consistency and Avoiding Burnout

5. The Impact of Fitness on Mental and Physical Health Part II: Embracing a Vegan Lifestyle

6. Understanding Vegan Nutrition: Macros, Micros, and Myth-Busting 7. Transitioning to a Vegan Diet: Practical Tips and Common Challenges 8. Supplements and Vegan Diets: What You Need to Know

Part III: Recipes and Meal Plans

9. Vegan Recipes for Active Lifestyles: Pre and Post Workout Meals 10. Weekly Meal Plans: From Quick Fixes to Elaborate Dishes 11. Seasonal and Local Eating: Maximizing Flavor and Sustainability Part IV: Veganism and Athletic Performance

12. Optimizing Your Diet for Performance: The Vegan Athlete 13. Case Studies: Success Stories of Vegan Athletes

Part V: Sustainable Practices

14. Sustainable Fitness Gear: Choosing Ethically Produced Equipment and Clothing 15. Reducing Your Environmental Footprint: Practical Steps for Everyday Life Part VI: Mindfulness and Well-being

16. Integrating Mindfulness into Fitness: Benefits and Techniques 17. Yoga and Meditation for Athletes: Enhancing Flexibility and Focus Conclusion

18. Living the Lumeim Way: Bringing It All Together

19. Building a Community: How to Connect with Like-Minded Individuals Appendices

•

Appendix A: Resources for Further Reading

•

Appendix B: Glossary of Terms

•

Appendix C: How to Stay Updated with Lumeim

Introduction: Welcome to Lumeim

Welcome to Lumeim, where every thread we weave and every product we create is designed to illuminate your path to fitness and well-being. At Lumeim, we believe that your workout attire and accessories should do more than just fit well—they should inspire, empower, and light up your journey towards health and fitness.

Our brand is founded on the principle that great design can transform your workout experience, making each session not just a routine but a step towards greater self-awareness and achievement.

Lumeim stands at the intersection of innovation and style, where each product is crafted to enhance visibility, focus, and performance.

In this book, we aim to extend the philosophy of our brand into every aspect of your fitness and wellness journey. We will share insights into developing a sustainable fitness routine, embracing a nutritious vegan diet, and integrating mindfulness into your daily life. Our goal is to support you in achieving a balanced and enlightened lifestyle that resonates with the core values of Lumeim: health, fitness, and sustainability.

As you turn each page, we invite you to explore not only our products but also the lifestyle and community that Lumeim fosters. Whether you are a seasoned athlete or just beginning your fitness journey, this book is your companion in discovering the brighter side of fitness—a journey lit with clarity, purpose, and innovation.

Join us as we delve into the Philosophy of Lumeim in the next section, where we will discuss how our ethos of health, fitness, and sustainability is woven into the very fabric of our products and practices.

Let's illuminate your fitness journey together, with Lumeim.

Philosophy of Lumeim: Ethos of Health, Fitness, and Sustainability At Lumeim, our philosophy extends beyond creating high-quality athletic apparel; it embodies a commitment to nurturing your health, invigorating your fitness endeavors, and fostering a sustainable environment. Our ethos is built on three foundational pillars: Health, Fitness, and Sustainability, each interwoven with our brand's DNA to not only inspire but also transform how you engage with your fitness lifestyle.

Health: Nourishing Body and Mind

Health is holistic. At Lumeim, we believe that true wellness encompasses both physical and mental health. Our products are designed to support your body's needs during workouts and recovery, ensuring comfort, functionality, and durability. But beyond the physical, we aim to empower you with knowledge and resources that foster mental resilience and well-being. This book will guide you through nutritional strategies, stress management techniques, and ways to harness the psychological benefits of a vegan diet and regular physical activity.

Fitness: More Than Just Exercise

Fitness at Lumeim is not just about vigorous workouts; it's about creating a lifestyle that encourages movement and improvement in all areas of life. Whether it's yoga, running, weightlifting, or casual jogging, our products are tailored to enhance every activity and support your performance goals. We advocate for a fitness routine that respects your body's limits while challenging you to expand them responsibly.

Through detailed workout plans, expert advice, and motivational stories, we'll help you find joy in the journey of becoming your fittest self.

Sustainability: A Commitment to the Planet

Sustainability is at the heart of everything we do. From the materials we choose to the production processes we employ, Lumeim is dedicated to minimizing environmental impact. Our commitment goes beyond our products—it's about promoting a lifestyle that values eco-conscious choices. In this book, you'll learn how integrating sustainable practices into your daily routine can be simple and impactful.

We'll explore topics such as choosing sustainable food options, reducing waste, and selecting eco-friendly fitness gear.

By adopting Lumeim's philosophy, you join a movement of individuals who are not only committed to personal health and fitness but are also advocates for a healthier planet. Our vision is to create a community where everyone feels empowered to make choices that illuminate their lives and the world around them.

In the next sections, we will delve deeper into practical applications of these philosophies, starting with foundational fitness and health strategies. Stay tuned to learn how to implement the Lumeim lifestyle seamlessly into your daily routine, ensuring that every step you take is illuminated by clarity, purpose, and conscious choice. Join us on this enlightening journey to a healthier, fitter, and more sustainable life.

Part I: Foundations of Fitness and Health 3. Getting Started with Fitness: Basics for Beginners to Advanced Embarking on a fitness journey can be exciting and daunting, regardless of whether you're a beginner or looking to enhance an established routine. At Lumeim, we understand that every fitness journey is unique, and our goal is to provide you with the foundational knowledge and tools necessary to ensure a successful and enjoyable path to better health and performance.

Understanding Your Fitness Level: Before diving into any workout regimen, it's crucial to assess your current fitness level. This evaluation should consider your physical capabilities, any health limitations, and your overall fitness goals. Such assessments can guide you in selecting the appropriate intensity and type of exercises that will yield the best results without risking injury.

Setting Realistic Goals: Goal setting is fundamental in keeping you motivated and on track. Start with clear, achievable goals that challenge you yet are within reach. Whether it's improving strength, endurance, flexibility, or weight loss, your goals should be Specific, Measurable, Achievable, Relevant, and Time-bound (SMART).

Creating a Balanced Routine: A well-rounded fitness regimen includes cardiovascular training, strength training, flexibility exercises, and balance training. Beginners might start with simple activities like walking, light jogging, or yoga, gradually increasing intensity and complexity as their fitness improves. For more advanced individuals, it's about diversifying workouts and incorporating higher intensity and resistance training to avoid plateaus and continue progress.

Equipment and Environment: Choosing the right equipment and environment can significantly enhance your workout experience. Lumeim's range of athletic wear is designed to support your body during various exercises, ensuring comfort and effectiveness. Additionally, creating a conducive workout space, whether at home or choosing the right gym, plays a crucial role in maintaining regular exercise habits.

Educational Resources and Guidance: Utilizing resources such as fitness apps, online tutorials, or personal trainers can provide guidance and structure, especially important for beginners. For those more advanced, workshops and specialized coaching can introduce new techniques and refine existing skills.

In this section, you'll find detailed workouts tailored to different fitness levels, expert tips on progressing safely, and motivational insights to keep you engaged every step of the way. Lumeim is here to light up your path to fitness, making each workout not just effective but a truly enlightening experience.

4. Developing a Sustainable Fitness Routine: Building Consistency and Avoiding Burnout Creating a fitness routine that is sustainable over the long term is key to achieving lasting health benefits. At Lumeim, we believe that a well-structured, adaptable fitness routine is essential not just for reaching physical goals but for fostering lifelong habits that promote overall well-being.

Consistency Over Intensity: One of the most common misconceptions in fitness is that more intense and frequent workouts yield better results. However, consistency is far more important than intensity. A moderate, regular workout schedule is more sustainable and less likely to lead to burnout or injury. It's important to find a rhythm that fits into your lifestyle and can be maintained over the long haul.

Variety in Your Routine: To keep your fitness routine engaging and effective, incorporate a variety of exercises. This not only prevents boredom but also ensures all muscle groups are worked and improves various aspects of fitness such as strength, endurance, flexibility, and balance. Alternating between different types of activities—such as weight training, cardio, yoga, and active recovery days—can keep the routine fresh and exciting.

Listen to Your Body: Paying attention to your body's signals is crucial. Overtraining can lead to burnout, decreased performance, and injury. Rest days are essential as they allow your muscles to recover and grow. If you feel tired or sore, it may be a sign to take it easy or focus on recovery techniques like stretching, massage, or light yoga.

Setting and Adjusting Goals: As you progress in your fitness journey, your goals will naturally evolve. Regularly reassess and adjust your goals to reflect your current fitness level, interests, and life circumstances. This dynamic approach keeps your routine aligned with what is motivating and achievable for you at any given time.

Community and Support: Engaging with a community or having a workout partner can greatly enhance your motivation and commitment. Lumeim encourages joining our community events, online forums, or local workout groups to share experiences, challenges, and successes. The support of others can be a powerful motivator and provides a network of accountability.

Tracking Progress: Using tools to track your progress, such as fitness apps, journals, or even simple tracking sheets, can provide you with concrete feedback on your performance and improvements. Celebrate milestones, no matter how small, as each step forward is a victory in your fitness journey.

In this section, you will find strategies to craft a personalized workout plan, tips on avoiding common pitfalls, and inspiration from community stories that highlight the joys and challenges of building a sustainable fitness routine.

With these principles, your fitness regimen will not only be a source of health and vitality but also a long-term, enjoyable part of your life.

5. The Impact of Fitness on Mental and Physical Health Physical fitness is integral to maintaining a healthy body and mind. At Lumeim, we emphasize the interconnected benefits of regular physical activity, which encompass not only the body's strength and endurance but also the mind's resilience and clarity. Here, we explore the extensive impact of fitness on both mental and physical health, supported by scientific research and anecdotal evidence from the Lumeim community.

Physical Health Benefits:

- Cardiovascular Health: Regular aerobic exercise, such as running, swimming, or cycling, strengthens the heart and improves circulation, significantly reducing the risk of cardiovascular diseases.

- Musculoskeletal Strength: Strength training exercises enhance muscle strength and bone density, crucial for overall body support and the prevention of osteoporosis.

- Weight Management: Engaging in physical activities helps to burn calories and regulate body weight, which is vital in preventing obesity-related diseases like type 2 diabetes.

- Enhanced Immunity: Regular exercise promotes a healthy immune system by rejuvenating the body's cells and systems.

Mental Health Benefits:

-

Mood Improvement: Physical activity triggers the release of endorphins, chemicals in the brain that act as natural painkillers and mood elevators, combating stress and depression.

•

Stress Reduction: Exercise reduces levels of the body's stress hormones, such as adrenaline and cortisol, while stimulating the production of endorphins.

•

Sleep Enhancement: Regular physical activity can help you fall asleep faster and deepen your sleep, crucial for overall mental health and cognitive function.

•

Increased Self-esteem: Achieving fitness goals often leads to improved self-esteem and self-worth, as physical achievements foster feelings of accomplishment.

Cognitive and Emotional Benefits:

•

Cognitive Function: Exercise improves cognitive function by increasing blood and oxygen flow to the brain, which is essential for the growth of neural connections and the overall health of brain cells.

•

Emotional Resilience: The challenges faced and overcome during exercise help build emotional strength, teaching individuals to manage adversity and recover from setbacks.

•

Enhanced Concentration: Regular physical activity helps sharpen concentration and extends periods of sustained mental effort, which is beneficial in personal and professional life.

Social and Lifestyle Benefits:

•

Community Building: Participating in group fitness activities can enhance social interaction and create bonds, contributing to a sense of belonging and community.

•

Lifestyle Enhancement: Regular exercise instills discipline and promotes a healthy lifestyle, influencing other areas such as dietary habits and mental health management.

Longevity:

•

Increased Lifespan: Studies have shown that regular exercise contributes to a longer lifespan by reducing the risk of developing chronic diseases and maintaining bodily functions.

Each benefit detailed above is a testament to the powerful role fitness plays in enhancing quality of life. At Lumeim, we integrate these principles into our products and practices, ensuring that our community not only achieves their physical goals but also enjoys robust mental health and a vibrant social life. Our commitment is to guide and support you through every step of your fitness journey, making it a rich and rewarding experience.

Having explored the profound effects of fitness on both mental and physical health, let's delve into the essentials of adopting and maintaining a vegan lifestyle in the next part of our book. This will include nutritional advice, practical diet tips, and the benefits of plant-based eating for both health and the environment.

6. Understanding Vegan Nutrition: Macros, Micros, and Myth-Busting Adopting a vegan lifestyle can be a transformative journey not only for your health but also for the environment. In this section, we'll delve deep into the essentials of vegan nutrition, focusing on macro and micronutrients, and debunk some common myths to ensure you have a balanced and informed approach to vegan eating.

Macro and Micronutrients in a Vegan Diet:

-

Proteins: Often a major concern for those considering a vegan diet, protein is abundant in plant sources like legumes, beans, lentils, tofu, and tempeh. These sources provide essential amino acids necessary for muscle repair and growth.

-

Fats: Healthy fats are vital for brain health and energy. Avocados, nuts, seeds, and oils like olive and flaxseed provide omega-3 and omega-6 fatty acids, crucial for maintaining heart health and reducing inflammation.

-

Carbohydrates: Carbohydrates are the body's primary energy source. Whole grains, fruits, and vegetables are excellent sources of complex carbohydrates, fiber, and a plethora of vitamins and minerals.

-

Micronutrients: Certain micronutrients require attention in a vegan diet, including Vitamin B12, Vitamin D, iron, calcium, and zinc. Fortified foods and supplements can help manage these needs effectively.

Myth-Busting:

•

Protein Deficiency: The myth of protein deficiency in vegan diets is pervasive but largely unfounded if a well-rounded and diverse diet is maintained.

•

Calcium and Bone Health: While dairy products are known for their calcium content, many plant-based options like broccoli, kale, and fortified plant milks also offer ample calcium.

•

Iron Absorption: Plant-based iron sources are abundant but are better absorbed when consumed with Vitamin C-rich foods, debunking the myth that vegans are iron-deficient.

Practical Tips for Transitioning:

•

Start Slow: Gradually incorporate more plant-based meals into your diet rather than making an abrupt shift, which can be sustainable and less overwhelming.

•

Learn to Read Labels: Understanding product labels can help you make informed choices about vegan products and avoid hidden animal-derived ingredients.

•

Experiment with Recipes: Explore the diversity of vegan cooking by trying new recipes that replicate your favorite non-vegan dishes with plant-based ingredients.

Incorporating these nutritional guidelines will help you maintain a healthy, balanced vegan diet that supports your fitness and overall well-being. Lumeim supports this journey with nutritional advice tailored to enhancing athletic performance and ensuring that your body receives the fuel it needs to excel.

Next, let's explore some delicious vegan recipes tailored for active lifestyles, which will help you integrate these nutritional concepts practically into your daily life.

7. Vegan Recipes for Active Lifestyles: Pre and Post Workout Meals A well-planned vegan diet can fuel the highest levels of fitness performance and recovery. In this section, we provide a selection of recipes designed specifically for active individuals. These recipes ensure that you receive optimal nutrition for energy before workouts and recovery afterward, all while adhering to a vegan lifestyle.

Pre-Workout Meals:

•

Banana and Almond Butter Toast: Quick to prepare and packed with good carbohydrates and proteins. The bananas provide natural sugars for energy, and almond butter adds a dose of healthy fats and protein to keep you satiated and energetic.

•

Oatmeal with Mixed Berries and Chia Seeds: Oats are an excellent source of sustained energy, and berries add antioxidants that help reduce workout-induced oxidative stress. Chia seeds provide omega-3 fatty acids and protein.

•

Smoothie Bowl: Blend a mix of spinach, a banana, a handful of blueberries, plant-based protein powder, and almond milk. This smoothie is light yet energizing, perfect for a pre-workout boost.

•

Tofu and Veggie Stir-Fry over Brown Rice: Tofu is a great source of plant-based protein, essential for muscle repair. Combine it with a variety of vegetables for nutrients and fiber, served over brown rice for a wholesome meal.

•

Lentil Soup with Sweet Potatoes and Kale: Lentils are rich in protein and fiber, aiding in muscle recovery and satiety. Sweet potatoes provide complex carbohydrates necessary for replenishing muscle glycogen, while kale adds a nutrient-dense component.

•

Quinoa Salad with Black Beans, Avocado, and Lime Dressing: Quinoa and black beans make this dish a protein powerhouse. Avocado provides healthy fats, and a zesty lime dressing adds a refreshing flavor while contributing Vitamin C

for immune support.

Each recipe is designed not just for taste but also to enhance athletic performance and recovery, aligning with the Lumeim philosophy of promoting health, fitness, and sustainability. These meals are easy to prepare, ensuring that maintaining a vegan diet is convenient and enjoyable.

Now that we have shared some practical and nutritious vegan recipes tailored for active lifestyles, let's continue to the next section where we will offer comprehensive weekly meal plans. These plans will help you effortlessly integrate these meals into your routine, supporting your health and fitness goals with every dish.

8. Weekly Meal Plans: From Quick Fixes to Elaborate Dishes
Creating a structured meal plan can significantly ease the transition to a vegan diet, ensuring that you consistently receive a balanced intake of nutrients while also catering to your active lifestyle. In this section, we provide detailed weekly meal plans that feature a variety of dishes, from quick fixes for busy days to more elaborate meals for when you have more time to enjoy cooking.

Week 1: Introduction to Vegan Eating

-

Monday:

-

Breakfast: Overnight oats with almond milk, chia seeds, and fresh berries.

-

Lunch: Chickpea salad with cucumbers, tomatoes, red onion, and a tahini dressing.

-

Dinner: Vegan chili made with kidney beans, quinoa, and a variety of vegetables.

-

Tuesday:

-

Breakfast: Green smoothie with spinach, mango, banana, and flaxseeds.

-

Lunch: Avocado toast with crushed red pepper and lime.

•

Dinner: Stuffed bell peppers with brown rice and black beans.

Week 2: High-Protein Focus for Active Individuals

•

Monday:

•

Breakfast: Tofu scramble with spinach, mushrooms, and onions.

•

Lunch: Lentil soup with carrots, celery, and onions.

•

Dinner: Tempeh stir-fry with broccoli, bell peppers, and soy sauce over brown rice.

•

Tuesday:

•

Breakfast: Peanut butter and banana smoothie with oat milk and vegan protein powder.

•

Lunch: Quinoa salad with edamame, carrots, cucumber, and a sesame dressing.

•

Dinner: Black bean tacos with avocado, salsa, and lettuce.

Week 3: Quick and Easy Vegan Meals

-

Monday:

-

Breakfast: Vegan yogurt with granola and a drizzle of agave syrup.

-

Lunch: Hummus and veggie wrap with spinach, bell pepper, and cucumber.

-

Dinner: Vegan pasta with tomato sauce and roasted vegetables.

-

Tuesday:

-

Breakfast: Fruit salad with a squeeze of lime and a sprinkle of mint.

-

Lunch: Vegan sushi rolls with avocado, cucumber, and carrot.

-

Dinner: Sweet potato and black bean burger with a side of steamed green beans.

Each meal plan is designed to provide a balance of macronutrients, ensuring that you get the proteins, fats, and carbohydrates needed to support your fitness activities and overall health. The recipes also include a variety of micronutrients that are vital for maintaining body functions and promoting recovery and muscle growth.

These meal plans not only make it easier for you to stay on track with a healthful, vegan diet but also ensure that your meals are aligned with the Lumeim brand's values of health, fitness, and sustainability. By following these plans, you'll enjoy delicious, nourishing meals that support your active lifestyle and contribute to a healthier planet.

Having established a solid foundation of nutritious vegan eating, let's move forward to explore how a vegan diet can be optimized specifically for athletic performance in the next section.

9. Optimizing Your Diet for Performance: The Vegan Athlete For athletes, nutrition plays a critical role in performance, recovery, and overall health. A vegan diet, when properly planned, can meet all the nutritional needs of athletes, from amateur fitness enthusiasts to elite competitors. In this section, we'll explore how to optimize a vegan diet for athletic performance, focusing on key nutrients and timing meals for maximum benefit.

Key Nutrients for Vegan Athletes:

•

Protein: Essential for muscle repair and growth, vegan athletes should focus on consuming a variety of protein sources such as lentils, chickpeas, tofu, tempeh, and quinoa. Plant-based protein powders can also be a helpful supplement around workouts.

•

Carbohydrates: The primary source of energy for athletes, carbs should be consumed in sufficient quantities to fuel workouts and aid in recovery. Sources like sweet potatoes, oats, fruits, and whole grains are optimal for sustained energy.

●

Fats: Healthy fats are crucial for hormonal health and energy. Nuts, seeds, avocados, and plant oils should be included daily to ensure adequate intake.

●

Iron: Plant-based diets can be high in non-heme iron, which is less readily absorbed by the body. Combining iron-rich foods like spinach and lentils with vitamin C-rich foods such as oranges or bell peppers can enhance absorption.

●

Calcium and Vitamin D: Important for bone health, these nutrients can be sourced from fortified plant milks and juices, as well as from dietary supplements if necessary.

Meal Timing for Peak Performance:

●

Pre-Workout Meals: Consume a carbohydrate-rich snack or meal 1-2 hours before exercise to top up energy stores. A small amount of protein can help prevent muscle breakdown.

Example: A banana with a small handful of almonds.

●

Post-Workout Recovery: After exercising, the focus should be on replenishing energy stores with carbohydrates and providing protein for muscle repair. A ratio of 3:1 carbs to protein within 30 minutes of finishing your workout can significantly aid recovery. Example: A smoothie made with vegan protein powder, a date, and a handful of berries.

Hydration: Maintaining hydration is essential for athletic performance and recovery. Athletes should drink water consistently throughout the day and adjust intake based on the intensity of exercise and environmental conditions.

Supplementation: Depending on individual needs and the specific demands of their sport, vegan athletes might consider supplements such as B12, vitamin D, omega-3 fatty acids (from algae sources), and possibly iron. It's advisable to consult with a healthcare provider to tailor supplementation appropriately.

Practical Tips for Vegan Athletes:

- Track Nutrient Intake: Using food tracking apps to monitor nutrient intake can be helpful, especially when transitioning to a vegan diet.

- Experiment with Foods and Timing: Each athlete is unique, so it's important to experiment with different foods and timing to see what works best for your body and your sport.

- Consult with a Dietitian: Working with a dietitian who specializes in vegan sports nutrition can provide customized advice and adjustments based on training demands.

By focusing on these nutritional strategies, vegan athletes can perform at their best, recover more efficiently, and maintain an ethical diet that aligns with their personal and environmental values.

Now that we have covered how to optimize a vegan diet for athletic performance, we are ready to explore the broader implications of sustainable practices within and beyond the diet.

Part V: Sustainable Practices

10. Sustainable Fitness Gear: Choosing Ethically Produced Equipment and Clothing In aligning with the core values of Lumeim, which emphasize sustainability alongside health and fitness, it's crucial to consider the environmental impact of all aspects of our fitness lifestyle, including the gear and apparel we choose. This section explores how to make informed, ethical choices in fitness gear and clothing, supporting not only personal health but also the health of our planet.

Materials and Production:

- Eco-Friendly Materials: Opt for fitness gear and apparel made from sustainable materials such as organic cotton, bamboo, recycled polyester, and Tencel. These materials are produced with lower environmental impact, reducing water usage and chemical outputs.

- Ethical Manufacturing: Support brands that are transparent about their manufacturing processes and adhere to fair labor practices. This ensures that the products are not only environmentally friendly but also socially responsible.

- Durability and Quality: Choosing high-quality items that last longer means purchasing less frequently, thereby reducing waste and demand for resources. Look for guarantees and reviews that attest to the product's durability.

Recycling and Upcycling:

- Recycling Old Gear: Many companies offer recycling programs for old gear, turning them into new products. Participating in these programs helps reduce landfill waste.

•

Upcycling: Consider upcycling older athletic wear for other uses, such as turning t-shirts into cleaning rags or repurposing sneakers for gardening.

Minimizing Impact:

•

Reducing Packaging: Choose products with minimal packaging, or packaging made from recycled or biodegradable materials. This reduces the waste associated with your fitness purchases.

•

Carbon Footprint: Consider the shipping and transportation of fitness products.

Buying locally can reduce carbon emissions associated with long-distance transportation.

Supporting Sustainable Brands:

•

Research and Choose Wisely: Invest time in researching brands that are committed to sustainability. Support those that align with your values and are making tangible efforts to improve their practices.

•

Certifications: Look for certifications like Fair Trade, Bluesign, Oeko-Tex, or B Corp, which indicate high standards of environmental and social responsibility.

By adopting these practices, you contribute to a more sustainable fitness culture that prioritizes long-term ecological health alongside physical health. Lumeim is committed to guiding and supporting you in making these choices, enhancing your fitness journey while also caring for the environment.

In the next section, we will explore additional ways to reduce your environmental footprint in everyday life, further expanding on the sustainable practices that form an integral part of the Lumeim ethos.

11. Reducing Your Environmental Footprint: Practical Steps for Everyday Life Embracing sustainability goes beyond choosing the right fitness gear; it involves integrating eco-friendly practices into all facets of daily life. At Lumeim, we encourage a lifestyle that minimizes environmental impact while promoting health and well-being. This section provides practical tips for reducing your environmental footprint in various aspects of everyday living.

Energy Consumption:

•

Green Energy Solutions: Opt for renewable energy sources if available, such as solar or wind power for your home. This reduces reliance on fossil fuels and lowers greenhouse gas emissions.

•

Energy Efficiency: Implement energy-saving measures at home, like using LED lighting, energy-efficient appliances, and smart thermostats. These small changes can significantly reduce your overall energy consumption.

Waste Reduction:

•

Reduce, Reuse, Recycle: Apply the three Rs rigorously in your daily routine. Minimize waste by choosing reusable options over single-use products, such as cloth shopping bags, reusable water bottles, and silicone food storage bags.

- Composting: Start composting kitchen scraps and yard waste to reduce landfill contribution and create nutrient-rich soil for gardening, which in turn can support local flora and fauna.

Water Conservation:

- Efficient Water Use: Install low-flow faucets and showerheads to reduce water usage. Be mindful of water use in daily activities, like turning off the tap while brushing teeth or fixing leaks promptly.

- Sustainable Landscaping: Opt for native plants in your garden, which require less water and maintenance. Consider rainwater harvesting systems to irrigate your garden, further reducing your potable water usage.

Transportation and Travel:

- Eco-Friendly Commuting: Whenever possible, walk, bike, or use public transportation to reduce carbon emissions. For longer distances, consider carpooling or driving an electric or hybrid vehicle.

- Mindful Travel: Choose travel options that minimize environmental impact. Support eco-friendly accommodations and activities that respect local ecosystems and communities.

Mindful Consumption:

-

Support Local and Organic: Purchase locally-produced and organic foods when possible. This supports local farmers, reduces transportation emissions, and minimizes chemical use in agriculture.

•

Conscious Shopping: Be thoughtful about purchases. Buy from companies that are transparent about their supply chains and committed to sustainable practices. Consider the lifecycle of the items you buy, choosing those that are made to last.

By adopting these sustainable practices, you can significantly reduce your environmental footprint, contributing to a healthier planet. Lumeim is dedicated to empowering you to make these changes, offering support and resources to help integrate these actions into your life seamlessly.

Having explored comprehensive strategies for sustainable living, let's continue our journey by examining how mindfulness and well-being are integrated into the Lumeim lifestyle, enhancing not only personal health but also our collective environmental responsibility.

Part VI: Mindfulness and Well-being

12. Integrating Mindfulness into Fitness: Benefits and Techniques
At Lumeim, we recognize that physical health and mental well-being are profoundly interconnected.

Mindfulness—the practice of maintaining a nonjudgmental state of heightened or complete awareness of one's thoughts, emotions, or experiences on a moment-to-moment basis—can greatly enhance the effectiveness of physical fitness routines and overall life satisfaction. This section explores how integrating mindfulness into your fitness regimen and daily activities can lead to greater mental clarity, improved physical performance, and enhanced well-being.

Benefits of Mindfulness in Fitness:

•

Enhanced Focus and Concentration: Mindfulness helps in focusing on the present moment, which can enhance the quality of workouts by improving concentration on form and execution of movements.

•

Stress Reduction: Regular mindfulness practice can lower stress levels, not only during workouts but throughout daily activities, helping to prevent burnout and improve overall mental health.

•

Increased Body Awareness: Mindfulness increases body awareness, which can lead to better posture, improved technique, and reduced risk of injury during exercise.

•

Emotional Equilibrium: Engaging in mindful exercise can help manage emotions effectively, aiding in quicker emotional recovery and promoting a balanced mood.

Techniques for Integrating Mindfulness into Fitness Routines:

•

Mindful Breathing: Focus on your breath during workouts. This can be as simple as being aware of the inhalation and exhalation during each exercise. Mindful breathing not only regulates the breath but also increases oxygen supply to the muscles, improving performance.

•

Body Scan: Start or end your workouts with a body scan— gradually focusing on each part of your body, acknowledging sensations without judgment. This practice enhances connection with your body and can highlight areas needing attention or recovery.

•

Yoga and Tai Chi: Incorporate mindful practices such as yoga or tai chi into your routine.

These disciplines combine physical movement with breath control and mental focus, embodying the essence of mindfulness in movement.

•

Set Intentional Goals: Before beginning your workout, set an intention. This could be a focus on gratitude for the ability to move, a dedication to improving health, or simply being present throughout the session.

Mindfulness Throughout the Day:

•

Mindful Eating: Apply mindfulness to eating by focusing on the flavors, textures, and sensations of your food. This practice can enhance digestion and satisfaction with meals.

•

Active Listening: Engage fully in conversations by focusing completely on the other person, helping to improve relationships and communication.

•

Regular Meditation: Dedicate time for regular meditation, even if it's just a few minutes a day. Meditation can reduce stress, increase focus, and contribute to a greater sense of peace and well-being.

By embracing mindfulness, you can transform not only your fitness routine but also your overall approach to life. The benefits extend beyond the gym, improving interactions, work performance, and personal relationships. Lumeim champions these practices as essential components of a holistic approach to health and fitness, ensuring that our community members lead enriched, balanced, and fulfilling lives.

Having explored the enriching integration of mindfulness into both fitness and everyday life, we now conclude our journey through this book, aiming to consolidate the lifestyle lessons and insights shared.

Conclusion: Living the Lumeim Way

As we conclude our journey through this comprehensive guide on health, fitness, and a sustainable, mindful lifestyle, it's important to reflect on how the principles and practices outlined in this book are more than just guidelines—they are the foundation of a transformative way of life. The Lumeim way is about enlightening your path to wellness, empowering you with knowledge, and inspiring a commitment to health and sustainability that resonates deeply and sustainably.

Consolidating Lifestyle Lessons:

•

Holistic Health: We've explored how integrating physical activity, a nutritious vegan diet, and mindfulness can significantly enhance both mental and physical health.

The Lumeim way is about embracing these elements cohesively, ensuring they complement and enhance one another.

•

Sustainability as a Core Value: From choosing sustainable fitness gear to adopting eco-friendly daily practices, we've seen how sustainability can extend into all facets of our lives. This commitment is not only good for our health but essential for the health of our planet.

•

Community and Support: Throughout this guide, the importance of community has been emphasized. Connecting with like-minded individuals can provide the motivation and support needed to maintain and grow in this lifestyle.

Future Directions for Living the Lumeim Way:

•

Continued Learning and Growth: Health and fitness are dynamic fields with new research and trends continually emerging. Staying informed and open to learning will ensure that your practices remain effective and relevant.

•

Expanding Community Engagement: As you grow in your journey, consider leading by example and helping others. Engaging more deeply with the Lumeim community through events, forums, or social media can enrich your experience and spread the positive impact.

•

Personal Reflection and Adaptation: Regularly reflect on your goals, practices, and well-being to ensure they continue to align with your evolving needs and aspirations.

Adaptation is key to sustained engagement and satisfaction.

Closing Thoughts:

Living the Lumeim way is an ongoing commitment to yourself and the world around you.

It's a promise to pursue health, fitness, and sustainability with enthusiasm and responsibility. As you close this book, remember that each step you take in this direction not only improves your own life but also makes a difference in the larger tapestry of our shared environment.

Thank you for choosing to embark on this journey with us. We hope this guide serves as a beacon, illuminating your path to a brighter, healthier, and more sustainable future.

Here's to shining bright in all your endeavors—both on and off the mat.

Appendices

Appendix A: Resources for Further Reading

To continue your journey with Lumeim and deepen your understanding of health, fitness, and sustainability, we recommend the following resources. These books, websites, and articles provide valuable insights and extended knowledge that can help you further explore the principles discussed in this book.

Books:

1.

"How Not to Die" by Michael Greger - An in-depth look at the nutritional science behind how diet can prevent and reverse disease.

2.

"Eating Animals" by Jonathan Safran Foer - Explores the moral and environmental implications of our food choices.

3.

"The Blue Zones" by Dan Buettner - Investigates the world's longest-lived people and their secrets to health and longevity.

Websites:

1.

NutritionFacts.org - A non-profit resource that provides free updates on the latest in nutrition research via bite-sized videos.

2.

No Meat Athlete - A website dedicated to plant-based nutrition for athletes, offering meal plans, podcasts, and coaching.

3.

EcoWatch - Provides information on environmental issues that affect health, the planet's health, and solutions including sustainable practices.

Articles:

1.

"The Impact of a Plant-Based Diet on Fitness" - An article that explores how athletes can maintain peak performance on a vegan diet.

2.

"Sustainable Fashion 101: What You Need to Know" - An overview of sustainable fashion, why it matters, and how you can make more environmentally friendly clothing choices.

3.

"Mindfulness in the Age of Complexity" - Discusses how mindfulness practices can reduce stress and improve quality of life in today's fast-paced world.

These resources are curated to support your continuous learning and application of a health-conscious, environmentally aware lifestyle.

Appendix B: Glossary of Terms

This glossary defines key terms used throughout the book, aiding in your understanding of concepts related to health, fitness, veganism, and sustainability.

•

Aerobic Exercise: Any form of exercise that requires pumping of oxygenated blood by the heart to deliver oxygen to working muscles.

•

Micronutrients: Vitamins and minerals that organisms need in small amounts to orchestrate a range of physiological functions.

•

Plant-Based Diet: A diet consisting mostly or entirely of foods derived from plants, including vegetables, grains, nuts, seeds, legumes, and fruits, and with few or no animal products.

•

Sustainability: Avoidance of the depletion of natural resources in order to maintain an ecological balance.

•

Mindfulness: The practice of being aware of your body, mind, and feelings in the present moment, thought to create a feeling of calm.

Appendix C: How to Stay Updated with Lumeim

Staying connected with Lumeim means you'll never miss out on the latest updates, events, and innovations. Here's how you can stay informed and engaged:

•

Newsletter: Subscribe to our monthly newsletter via our website to receive updates on new products, special offers, and events.

•

Social Media: Follow Lumeim on platforms like Instagram, Facebook, and Twitter for daily inspiration, live sessions, and community stories.

•

Blog: Visit our blog for weekly posts on fitness tips, vegan recipes, and sustainable living practices.

•

Community Events: Participate in community workouts, webinars, and eco-friendly initiatives organized by Lumeim to connect with like-minded individuals and learn from experts.

By utilizing these resources and staying connected, you ensure that you are always at the forefront of innovations in health, fitness, and sustainability with Lumeim.

With these appendices, you have additional tools and information at your disposal to continue exploring and deepening your understanding of the principles laid out in this book. Whether through further reading, clear definitions, or staying engaged with the Lumeim community, your journey towards a healthier, more sustainable lifestyle is well-supported.